Make Her Orgasm Again and Again

48 Simple Tips & Tricks to Give Her Mind-Blowing, Explosive, Full-Body Orgasm After Orgasm, Night After Night

Elizabeth Cramer
Copyright© 2014 by Elizabeth Cramer

Copyright© 2014 Elizabeth Cramer

All Rights Reserved.

Warning: The unauthorized reproduction or distribution of this copyrighted work is illegal. No part of this book may be scanned, uploaded or distributed via internet or other means, electronic or print without the author's permission. Criminal copyright infringement without monetary gain is investigated by the FBI and is punishable by up to 5 years in federal prison and a fine of $250,000. (http://www.fbi.gov/ipr/). Please purchase only authorized electronic or print editions and do not participate in or encourage the electronic piracy of copyrighted material.

Publisher: Living Plus Healthy Publishing

ISBN-13: 978-1495293382

ISBN-10: 1495293386

Disclaimer

The Publisher has strived to be as accurate and complete as possible in the creation of this book. While all attempts have been made to verify information provided in this publication, the Publisher assumes no responsibility for errors, omissions, or contrary interpretation of the subject matter herein. Any perceived slights of specific persons, peoples, or organizations are unintentional.

This book is not intended for use as a source of legal, business, accounting or financial advice. All readers are advised to seek services of competent professionals in the legal, business, accounting, and finance fields.

The information in this book is not intended or implied to be a substitute for professional medical advice, diagnosis or treatment. All content contained in this book is for general information purposes only. Always consult your healthcare provider before carrying on any health program.

Table of Contents

Introduction 5

Part I: 21 Things You Must Know About Female Orgasm 7

    1. The vast majority of women are capable of having orgasms 7

    2. Only 25% of women have orgasms from regular intercourse alone 10

    3. You can have an orgasm and not know it 13

    4. An orgasm is a reflex 16

    5. There is no difference between vaginal and clitoral orgasms 21

    6. Female orgasms are faster than you think 24

    7. (For Her) Female orgasms happen in a series of short bursts 27

    8. Females do sometimes ejaculate 29

    9. (For Her) Lack of orgasm is not about relationship 33

10. (For Her) You can push yourself over the edge 36

11. The key to the end is the beginning 39

12. Orgasms were once prescribed to promote mental health 42

13. (For Her) You cannot get addicted to your vibrator 45

14. The G-Spot isn't really a thing 49

15. (For Her) Fantasy is required 52

16. (For Her) The best way to have an orgasm is to stop trying to have an orgasm 55

17. (For Her) The best time to have an orgasm is at the beginning of sex 58

18. Position matters 61

19. There is no magical pill for orgasm 65

20. Orgasm is not a sign of sexual experience or maturity 68

21 Orgasm has a purpose 69

Part II: 27 Techniques to Give Her Mind Blowing Pleasure 71

Foreplay 73

1. Take Your Time 73

   2. Start from Afar 75

   3. Play the Brain Game 77

   4. Wine to Water 79

   5. Wild Whispers 81

   6. Kiss Her Cares Away 83

   7. Copious Compliments 85

Techniques 87

   8. Who's On First 87

   9. Shoot for Two 89

   10. Save the Best for Last 91

   11. Never Try Dry 93

   12. Play in the Zone 95

   13. Multitask 97

   14. Look Her in the Eye 98

   15. Rock Concert 100

   16. Waiting is the Hardest Part 102

   17. The 90 Second Window 104

   18. Steady as She Blows 106

   19. Luscious Lips 108

   20. Light as a Feather 110

   21. Plug In 112

Positions 115

22. Go Against the Grain 115

23. Take her to the Top while on the Bottom
.... 117

24. Who Let The Dogs Out? 119

25. Do the Twist 121

26. Pillow talk 123

27. Use the CAT 125

Conclusion 127

Introduction

You've been thinking about her all day. Over and over in your mind you've been imagining the two of you making love tonight. You don't just want the evening to be a good experience. It needs to be a great experience for both of you. Searching your thoughts for the best wine to select or the right words to say, it dawns on you that the way to make the night memorable for you both is to ensure it ends with her having an explosive orgasm that rocks her world and shows you are an attentive and amazing lover. If that's the case, this guide is for you.

Mysterious, explosive, transcendent, hot, joyous, pulsing, out-of-control release; no matter how you describe it, orgasm is a one-of-a-kind experience. Every woman is a little different in how she feels it, and how she feels about it. Yet, this unique and supremely pleasurable moment is one of the most sought-after and misunderstood in our sexual lives.

This guide is divided into two parts. "*Part I: 21 Things You Must Know About Female Orgasm*" is the "what" and "*Part II: 27 Techniques to Give Her Mind Blowing Pleasure*" is the "how to." Although the target audience is men, women can also benefit from the information in this guide. Sections that are devoted to women readers are designated with "*For Her*" in titles. Men are recommended to read these sections as well as they help you get a full picture of female orgasm.

It's time to understand the magic moment, explode some myths, and get some tips on creating, sustaining and enjoying the outstanding "O."

Part I: 21 Things You Must Know About Female Orgasm

1. The vast majority of women are capable of having orgasms

One of the reasons so few women know or understand the scientific and social realities of orgasms is the relative silence in our culture on this topic. You can talk about a lot of things with friends in public or at a private picnic and somehow the subject of orgasms and who has them isn't one that comes up a lot. That leaves many in the dark about who is having the big O and who isn't. So, the myth prevails (particularly among women who have not had an orgasm) that there are a lot of women who simply "can't have them" and don't experience any sort of outward sign of their climax.

The opposite is true.

Sexologists from the American Gynecological and Obstetrics Association maintain that approximately 90% of women are capable of having orgasms. This number stands in direct contrast to the myths that orgasm is a culmination experience for only a few women. Why is it that so many women are capable of having orgasms but we think it's an exclusive club? Just because you CAN have one, doesn't mean you have.

The old theory is that women who are not capable of having an orgasm are "anorgasmic." There are two known types of what is described as anorgasmia: Primary Anorgasmia (the woman has never had an orgasm) and Secondary Anorgasmia (the woman had orgasms in the past but is no longer experiencing them).

The new understanding is that only 10% of women actually suffer from Anorgasmia. The majority of women who have never had an orgasm are now referred to as "pre-orgasmic" (they can have an orgasm; they just haven't had one yet) and women who seemed to have "stopped" having orgasms are referred to medical practitioners to look for the cause of the change in their sexual expression. Many women who stop having orgasms, even though their sexual life has not changed, are suffering from a medical problem or a medicinal side-effect.

Now that we don't believe women just "don't have orgasms" anymore, there is an increased motivation for women who are pre-orgasmic to learn more about the wonderful O and ways they can learn to have one. Orgasmic experience and sexual release are within the grasp of many women, they just need a little knowledge and practice to get the ball rolling.

2. Only 25% of women have orgasms from regular intercourse alone

In cultures where women don't receive adequate sexual education or are encouraged to see sexual intercourse solely as an act intended for procreation and not pleasure, the common response is to have intercourse and wait to see if something "different" happens.

If you're just lying there thinking the magic will spontaneously start, you have a three in four chance of being disappointed. Only 25% of women have orgasms solely through participating in intercourse.

In order for a woman to have an orgasm a certain number of things have to happen (see item #4) and most of them don't happen through intercourse alone. In order to stimulate and build tension throughout the pelvic area most women need to experience more than the rocking and thrusting of a penis during intercourse.

Additional stimulation from your partner or yourself focused on her clitoral area, or pressure applied to the lower pelvic area is often required to build the level of tension required to facilitate a release. Approximately 50% of women can achieve orgasm through intercourse coupled with extra stimulation. The remaining 25% of women who experience orgasms do so without intercourse and achieve release solely through manual or oral stimulation.

Some women experience pain in the vaginal channel during regular intercourse that interferes with their bodies' ability to orgasm, and others are so focused on the rhythm and thrusting of intercourse they are not allowing their minds to aid in the reflexive action resulting in orgasm.

Anything that preoccupies her mind, such as pain, distraction or discomforting thoughts, is likely to keep her orgasm at bay. Manual or oral stimulation allows women a chance to focus her attention solely on the pleasure occurring at the moment and creates a likely scenario for release.

There is no "right" or "wrong" way to achieve an orgasm. Climaxing by means other than the act of intercourse (defined by sexologists as a "penis-in-vagina sexual experience") is the norm for most women. The more we teach women to understand what creates pleasure in their system and empower them to pursue those impulses the more satisfied women will be with their sexual experiences.

Although all women have the same physiological and biological attributes, every woman is built a little differently and will need to engage in some self-discovery to know exactly what will be the best method for her to reach climax.

3. You can have an orgasm and not know it

Not every woman who thinks of herself as anorgasmic or pre-orgasmic has, in fact, never experienced an orgasm. Women can have orgasms resulting in the same after-glow of pleasure and biochemical brain release but are not conscious that it is happening. There are several reasons this can happen.

Not only are all women different in their orgasmic experiences - orgasms themselves are different each time. Sometimes an orgasm can be a huge, mind-blowing, jaw dropping experience and other times an orgasm can be so small, fast, or lost in the whole sexual event that it happens and no one really notices.

An orgasmic wave or impulse can happen as quickly as 0.4 seconds. If she has a "low wave count" (1-3 waves) she is barely going to have time to register something is happening before it is over. Women who have these fast, tiny rockers often don't experience them but suddenly feel "finished" or "complete" in the sexual experience and begin to relax and feel contented.

Women who have experienced childhood abuse, a battering relationship or sexual trauma often "detach" during sexual experiences.

They go through the motions of having sex, and may even feel love or happiness based on the intimacy with their sexual partner. However, the more subtle or finer points of the sexual experience – particularly if they trigger a memory of a prior bad experience – often go undetected by conscious thought.

Trauma survivors use this level of detachment as a defense mechanism in order to get through the bad things that happened to them. Once they are in a good place it is hard to shut off the survival skill, and some have become so used to it they don't even realize it is happening. Only later, when a partner says something like, "Wow, you really enjoyed that one!" does a trauma survivor remember the convulsions or attributes of a climax having occurred.

It is not uncommon for a sexual trauma survivor to say she knows when she is having sex, but can't really remember or tell you much about what happened or how it felt. This phenomenon can be changed through interventional therapy, interactive communication with a sexual partner and time.

Physiologically, some women do not feel or experience contractions in the muscle of the pelvic floor. They experience vaginal or clitoral release but don't have the jolting motion and internal sensation that goes with it because their pelvic floor is not as responsive as the other muscles or areas involved. Without the hip thrusting motion and contraction a woman's orgasm feels more like a tingle or stinging pulse for a few seconds and she may not recognize it as an orgasm.

According to sex researchers, women who do not experience pelvic release often describe soreness or the inability to keep going sexually after the orgasm and are more likely to find continued stimuli after the climax painful or unwanted.

Frequently, without the pelvic floor contractions they believe they are not having "real orgasms" and think of themselves as anorgasmic. Kegel exercises and muscle awareness coupled with purposeful pelvic thrusts often help women experience a fuller and stronger orgasm in time.

4. An orgasm is a reflex

The Merriam-Webster Dictionary defines a reflex as "an automatic and often inborn response to a stimulus that involves a nerve impulse passing inward from a receptor to a nerve center and thence outward to an effector (as a muscle or gland)." That describes exactly the biomechanics of an orgasm.

So, if you're thinking an orgasm is the same thing as when your leg jerks because a doctor taps you below the knee with a hammer – you're right. But, orgasms are a more complex reflex, and frankly, more fun.

Orgasms start where everything else in your body does – your brain. Your body is made of nerves which travel through the spinal column (except for the vagus nerve) and connect to the brain. The genital area has a very high concentration of nerve endings. The female clitoris has the most of any body part on women– 8,000 nerve endings.

When those parts are stimulated, the impulse goes through the nerve up the spine to the brain. That explains why many women will say they feel an actual sensation "up their spine" when they are engaged in foreplay or become sexually aroused.

Four major nerves carry the signal to the brain during sex (making the event a nearly "full body" experience). The **hypogastric nerve** carries signals from the uterus and cervix. Also carrying a cervical signal along with vaginal nerve activity is the **pelvic nerve**. The **pudendal nerve** transmits impulses from the clitoris and the **vagus nerve** (the only nerve in the group that does not run through the spinal cord) carries different signals from the cervix, uterus and vagina.

During foreplay and early arousal all these nerves "check-in" with the brain and let it know something pleasurable is going on down below.

Many have heard of the "pleasure center" of the brain or the "reward circuit" – that's the part which experiences the release of certain brain chemicals and gives us a sense of pleasure or good feelings.

There are actually four parts of the brain, however, that make orgasms occur. The **amygdala** regulates emotion and helps the brain create and process feelings. The **VTA** (ventral tegmental area) releases dopamine (a pleasure-chemical) into the system while the **pituitary gland** releases beta-endorphins, oxytocin and vasopressin – stimulants which create feelings of bonding or trust, and actually decrease pain. The **nucleus accumbens** is responsible for controlling the dopamine release.

All those chemicals cause a reaction in the cerebellum, which functions to regulate muscle control and is what causes the involuntary muscle movement associated with orgasm.

As a timeline – orgasms work like this:

- Sexy thinking, foreplay and arousal cause two processes to start happening. The attention to the nerve endings sends signals to the brain and more blood begins to head toward the "affected area." An increase of endorphins and blood flow causes the vagina to secrete lubrication. The longer foreplay and arousal continue the more lubrication will be made.

- As sex goes forward, her blood increases in the pelvic area causing her breathing to speed up, heart rate to rise and nipples to become erect. All of this activity causes the lower vaginal opening to narrow which holds the penis more firmly, causing friction, and the upper part of the vaginal cavity to expand which allows space for the penis to thrust.

- The combination of friction, blood pressure, and nerve stimulation causes the muscles of the pelvic floor, vagina, clitoris and anus to tense (almost like a cramp).

- As the nerves send those signals to the brain the glands in the brain realize something must be done to release that tension (the brain processes sexual tension very similarly to the "fight or flight" response).

- The brain releases chemicals which affect the cerebellum and cause all the muscles to release at once in a small series of spasms resulting in momentary (a few seconds) loss of consciousness, muscle control, vocal control, and eyesight.

- After the tension is released, the chemicals secreted in the brain, particularly dopamine and serotonin, activate the pleasure center to create a sense of relaxation, pleasure and bonding.

- The cool down for the body, often called the "after-glow" allows the heart rate, blood flow, and breathing to go back to normal.

5. There is no difference between vaginal and clitoral orgasms

If you read a lot of women's magazines or shop online at sex toy stores you will hear a lot about the supposed difference between *vaginal* orgasms, *clitoral* orgasms, or *holistic* orgasms (a combination of the two).

Some women claim that clitoral orgasms are stronger and create an increased response. Others have suggested vaginal orgasms are somehow "deeper" and harder to achieve but "worth it" because of the prolonged pelvic thrusting involved in the "vaginal focus". Holistic or "total body" orgasms are often lifted up as the ultimate goal for an individual, only being trumped by a mutual holistic orgasm (when the male and female partner climax at the same time).

The sex toy market has furthered these claims by creating sex toys designed to *"hit the G spot"* (promoting a stronger vaginal response) or tickle the clitoris (toys with nubs or vibrating arms that touch the clitoris).

Popular toys such as the "rabbit vibrators" (or their many animal variations) are designed to concentrate stimulation in both areas at the same time, and vibrating anal plugs can be added to the mix in an attempt to inspire your body to complete the "whole package."

However, all of these claims miss a central truth. **There is absolutely no difference between a vaginal, clitoral or full-body orgasm.**

Why? Because all orgasms are full-body orgasms.

Dr. Betty Whipple in her book, *The G-Spot and Other Discoveries About Human Sexuality*, points out all orgasms come from the same bodily process (the relief of built up tension through autonomic response) and only differ in actual location.

If she has built up more tension in her pelvic floor (generally through thrusting or kegel exercises) or are using a vibrator concentrating more stimulation to the vaginal walls she is more likely to experience higher tension in the vaginal area and a more noticeable release.

If she is using a sexual position that allows more stimulation on the clitoris or indulging in manual stimulation while intercourse is occurring, more tension builds there, the nerves are activated and she feels a stronger release in that area.

That doesn't mean you need to go through your fun drawer and throw out all your electronic playmates. Every woman has different erogenous zones and each toy may hit a different part of her body. If the vibrator works for her and allows her stimulation in the spot where she is most likely to orgasm, keep it. However, don't feel like your sex life is somehow "lacking" or "not as good" as someone else's based on where her muscular release occurs.

All orgasms serve the same purpose and provide pleasure. The process is the same, and it's all good.

6. Female orgasms are faster than you think

Scientists and poets have it right: time is relative. When you are having a great time the hours can fly by feeling like a few minutes. When you are unhappy with what is going on or waiting for something good, time plods on lead shoes turning fifteen minutes into an eternity. It's no surprise, then, to realize that actual time an orgasm takes to work its magic is much faster than you can imagine.

Depending on the level of muscular tension and the time it takes her brain to create her release, the sum total of an orgasm lasts between 3 seconds (small tremor) to 15 seconds (long whopping "oh-my-gosh" kind of experience). In fact, by the time she registers an orgasm is happening, it is nearly over.

That's a good thing because at the increased heart and respiratory rates occurring during orgasm, we probably wouldn't live through one that was much longer. Women who sustain longer orgasms are far more likely to report soreness, oversensitivity or cramping during the afterglow phase.

Men, by contrast, have orgasms that last anywhere from 10 seconds to 30 seconds. For those who view that as somewhat unfair, time has its own balancing agent as well. The length and strength of women's orgasms remain about the same throughout the course of their whole lives. However, as men age their orgasms decrease in both length and strength of feeling.

Men's orgasms also become less frequent and less ejaculate is issued as the aging process continues. So, women might not hit the heights of a young man, but she will be rocking and rolling long after his peak is over.

There is no way for a woman to purposely expand the duration an orgasm will last, but she can do things to help with the strength and ease of a climax. Most women experience a range of lengths and sensations throughout their sex life. Circumstances can have an effect on that range. Women who abstain from sex long enough to build sexual frustration often find their orgasms are "sharp" and do not seem to last as long.

Sexologists believe that due to the length of muscle tension coupled with stimulus to the nerve endings, the body has become unaccustomed to feeling. It's similar to how someone touching your skin for the first time can make you jump, but if he touches you frequently you are less likely to react. More foreplay also leads to increased muscle tension which creates stronger sensations upon release.

A woman also reaches orgasm more quickly if she has already had one, and second orgasms tend to last longer in duration but have a weakened sensation.

If a woman wants to achieve an orgasm during intercourse, but usually doesn't, one thing she can try is to have her partner give her an orgasm before intercourse via oral or manual clitoral stimulation, then have intercourse. The second orgasm will come more easily and have a larger number of pulses.

However, when any nerve is over-stimulated the brain will "shut down" or mute the sensation via the release of oxytocin so muscle release and feelings you get from that will be less strong and satisfying.

Oxytocin and Vasopressin are both natural sleep agents; the more orgasms she has, no matter how long or short they seem, the more likely she is to get sleepy afterward.

7. (For Her) Female orgasms happen in a series of short bursts

All people are attracted to one of three sensations: floating, flying or falling. Women who like lounging on a pool mat or the sensation of being weightless are floaters. Flyers enjoy movement and the rush of wind in their face. Fallers - roller coaster riders and risk addicts - love the feeling of decompression and changes in altitude. Whichever sensation a woman is drawn to, the pattern of orgasm is made to fit right in.

Orgasm isn't just a one-time release characterized by fluttering body parts and arched backs. It actually happens as a series of waves or pulses. Each orgasmic wave lasts approximately 0.8 seconds. A "small" or "quick" orgasm consists of 1 – 3 waves. A longer or more sustained orgasm can have as many as 10 or 15 waves. The waves do not always come at perfectly timed intervals. The quicker the intervals, the stronger the sensation or pulse will seem.

The effect this has on the mind/body is very similar to the visualization of dropping a rock in a pond. The moment the rock is dropped clearly defined circles surround the entry spot. Those circles then stretch out becoming less well-defined the farther they get from the source until they dissipate into a larger body of water. This wave effect in women is what produces the feelings of relaxation and after-glow.

If you have an orgasm and jump up to get dressed as soon as you can see again, you'll be missing out on the best part of the experience. As the waves of relaxation pulse through the body, women feel warm, sensuous and experience the elevated sense of satisfaction caused by the dopamine and serotonin released as the waves go out from the pelvic area to encompass the whole body.

Some women find their sexual experiences to be lacking or describe their sex lives as uninspiring, even if they are having orgasms. It is likely they aren't giving their brain enough time to give them the full benefit of the experience.

Even though your orgasm itself is only seconds long, the after-glow can last up to 30 minutes with each wave of pleasure pulsing throughout your body. Make sure to take the time to experience the euphoria in order to sustain a sense of satisfaction in your sexual relationship.

8. Females do sometimes ejaculate

Perhaps one of the most hotly debated issues in the study of orgasms and women's sexuality as a whole, is the topic of female ejaculation. Physicians and researchers analyze the fluid that results from "female ejaculation" to determine the identity of the substance. Sexologists study claims, methods, and research to determine what is really happening, what effect it has on the sexual act, and how to cause this phenomenon in women who want it.

Feminists and philosophers argue about whether all this attention to the ejaculate is reducing a female's sexual experience so it will be on "par" with a male experience, thus robbing women of their unique role and value in sex. Film rating boards have commissioned research to determine what is happening so they can decide whether or not it is legal to permit a film featuring "female ejaculation" to be shown.

Even linguists have an opinion. Although the terms for the fluid that exits a female during orgasm (*ejaculate, gushing, squirting*) are used interchangeably in many circles, there really is a difference in those three terms and what they mean as a way of explaining what happens.

Ejaculate itself simply means to emit fluid from the body in a quick burst (a perfect description for what happens when men emit semen). However, in women the fluid doesn't spurt out in a few small jolts. Ejaculate is not a very good term to use for a woman's experience.

"Gushing" is used to describe the experience when excess fluid comes out of the vaginal opening during orgasm. If it sort of "bubbles" or "gushes" out, the fluid is excess vaginal lubrication or lubrication combined with pre-cum or semen deposited in the vaginal opening. What goes up must come down and what goes in will always come out.

Most women actually don't make enough vaginal lubrication which is why this doesn't happen to many women. However, if there is an abundance of fluid in the vaginal canal it will come out (or get "ejected") when the muscles of the pelvic floor contract during orgasm. If the fluid is not clear but curdled or smelly, it is possibly vaginal discharge and a trip to the gynecologist is needed.

Squirting, largely a fixture of porn movies and Tumblr gifs, is used to explain when a large volume of liquid comes squirting at a high rate of speed during orgasm. Chemical analysis of that fluid by sex researchers shows with great regularity that it is diluted urine. A small amount of urine sits at the base of the bladder and the combination of pressure (depending on what position is used for intercourse) and strong contractions siphons out the urine and pushes it out with some velocity. Because it is a residual amount, it doesn't always have a strong or pungent smell like urine expelled through normal means, but chemically, it's still urine.

Releasing fluid is not a sign that a woman's experience is better, deeper, more desirable or that a woman's lover is more skillful. It's simply a sign that the body has too much fluid and is expelling it as the muscles tighten and release. Remember that next time you hear a man proudly say, "I can make women squirt."

In Great Britain and many countries, there are film laws about showing things like urination in film. That's why the question of female ejaculation has been reviewed with some urgency. Many films have had to cut scenes featuring a female squirting in order for their films to be shown or distributed in certain countries if the content is presumed to be urine.

Feminist groups have argued successfully in court that a film claiming the scene is a shot of a female ejaculating demeans women and provides inaccurate sexual information. No matter what research ultimately discovers, this topic will be open for debate for some time to come.

9. (For Her) Lack of orgasm is not about relationship

Imagine you and your lover have settled into a long-term relationship. Your sex life has always been good. The norm for you as a couple is that you experience orgasms frequently, usually with extra stimulation, but not every time. Then you begin to notice it has been a while since you've experienced a climax.

When you talk about it with your partner he tells you he has noticed that as well and worries you aren't "into him" anymore. Suddenly, you begin to wonder about the same thing. The love is still there, sexual frequency is still there, trust and excitement are still part of your life – you just aren't achieving orgasm.

If you read women's magazines or relationship guides you're likely to believe something is happening to your relationship at some mysterious, deep, subconscious level. That simply would not be true. The sudden inability to have orgasms or lessoning of orgasms over time is almost never about the relationship (particularly if there is nothing you can pinpoint wrong with the relationship).

While it is understandably difficult to feel arousal if you are having sex that is unwanted or with someone you find repulsive, once you have ruled out those categories the lack of orgasm is largely explained by medical science, not relationship workshops. If you eat a sandwich your stomach is going to digest it, whether you like it or not, and whether you've eaten the same thing every day for a week or a year. Orgasm is the same way. There is no reason to believe that you have stopped loving or enjoying someone because you aren't having an orgasm. The system doesn't work like that.

Usually the reason for a change in orgasmic response is found in a medical condition (ranging in seriousness from slight to immediate) or medication a woman is taking. Diseases such as Multiple Sclerosis, Diabetic Neuropathy, or any kind of spinal cord injury can prevent the signals carried by the nerve endings to get to the brain. Other conditions such as a low-functioning thyroid, lymphatic system disorders, or basic hormonal changes due to menopause can also limit or change the amount of brain chemicals released. If you experienced regular orgasms and they suddenly stop happening, see your doctor for a complete check-up.

Medications also hinder or prevent sexual arousal or orgasms. Anti-depressants almost all have sexual side effects due to the changes they cause in serotonin release. While the changes in biochemical release help the brain manage depression, they also limit the brain's ability to chemically manage arousal and/or orgasm.

Muscle relaxers, such as Carisoprodol (Soma), Cyclobenzaprine (Flexeril) or oral steroids, keep the muscles from building the required tension that leads to orgasm. Even a consistent dosage of an NSAID can cause orgasms to happen less frequently or with less strength.

Other medications that inhibit orgasmic response are: anti-hypertensives (Thalitone, Synepril, Vivatec, etc.), anti-anxiety drugs, anti-psychotics (Lithium, Haldol, Geodone), cholesterol-reducing agents (Lipitor, Lanoxin), and advanced pain reducers (Morphine, Codeine, prescription Ibuprofen).

10. (For Her) You can push yourself over the edge

After a wonderful dinner out, an evening of sensual foreplay including chocolate covered strawberries and a massage, and a session of vigorous love making you find yourself on the edge of an orgasm. Your hips are rocking, mind is reeling, and heart is pounding. You feel the tension gripping every muscle you have. You are on the edge of the cliff and ready to jump off. Suddenly, your partner ejaculates and withdraws before you can achieve release. You clamp your jaws together to keep from issuing a loud sentence consisting mostly of profanity and fight the urge to cry, or slap him. But, there are things you can do to keep your train from stalling at frustration station.

First, take your focus off of him for a minute. Retreat into your mind. Imagine your intercourse is still going, or replace him with a mental scenario and a lover who won't stop until you are done. Keeping your brain engaged will keep the signals flowing.

Next, reach down with your own hand (if he won't do it for you) and continue to apply clitoral stimulation. What's important is that there is as little disruption in the flow of nerve signals as possible. Your brain doesn't have eyes, so if you are still thinking sexy thoughts (instead of the aforementioned slap) and your body is still sending signals reflecting stimulus, your brain will continue preparing for muscle release.

Finally, this is where all those kegel exercises pay off. Continue moving your hips and focus on your internal muscles. Tighten and release your pelvic floor muscles in a quick series of jolts. For example, tighten your pelvic floor muscle for 3 seconds then release for three seconds. If you aren't sure what your pelvic floor muscle is take some time prior to lovemaking to find it. The best way is to go to the bathroom and stop urination in midstream. That muscle you flexed to stop the flow is your pelvic floor. Stopping and starting urination is a great natural kegel exercise and will give you much more control over that muscle.

Between the stimuli applied to your clitoris, the feeling of the pelvic floor tightening and releasing and the fantasy going on in your head, you'll be jumping off that cliff in a few minutes (or less) and experiencing all the satisfaction you deserve. It is always nicer if your partner helps you conclude your climax, but if he doesn't then you'll have to follow that well-worn adage – "If you want something done right, you better do it yourself."

11. The key to the end is the beginning

A growing trend in Hollywood movies is to take a thriller or complex story and tell it out of sequence. In fact, some of the most highly acclaimed mysteries are told backwards where the end is revealed and the movie traces the story back to the beginning. If you want an orgasm that curls her toes and makes her see stars until she can't see anymore, you'll have to get her mind off the end and think about the beginning. When it comes to orgasms, arousal is the key.

Foreplay is one of those concepts that can't be defined scientifically (even though its results can be systematically measured) and can't be explained rationally. The word means something different to each person. For some, foreplay is a quick round of kissing followed by an inserted finger. It won't be a shock to learn the women in those situations are the least likely to have orgasms and the most likely to find their whole sexual relationship physically and emotionally unsatisfying.

On the other side of the spectrum are men who start the foreplay hours before with a tantalizing phone call before dinner, and continue throughout the evening offering touch, taste and experiences. Those couples tend to engage in intercourse for a longer period of time, increasing both the tension and the orgasm.

Arousal makes everything better because it involves the whole body in the orgasmic experience. Physical arousal in women increases blood flow to the muscle tissue, engorging sexual parts and making the nerve endings even more responsive to stimulus. Nipples, the vulva, and the clitoris all "check in" with the brain once a woman becomes aroused.

Arousal increases a woman's vaginal lubrication which allows for a more fluid and pleasurable experience, adding to the signals the engorged tissues are already sending. The combination of mental attraction and physical connection helps the brain regulate hormones and set up the perfect scenario for a long and strong "O". Arousal matters.

Not all kinds of foreplay are good for ensuring an orgasm, however. While a tray of wine and cheese is a romantic standard, you need to engage in that part a few hours before your intercourse begins. Alcohol is a depressant, and will limit the amount of pleasure hormones your brain sends out, as well as impair the brain's ability to read the sexual signals coming from the erogenous zones. Too much alcohol makes it harder for men to maintain an erection. In women, alcohol affects her ability to concentrate and tends to leave them sluggish, unresponsive and sleepy. Have any alcohol you plan for the evening at least 1 hour per ounce before your sexual interaction.

Similarly, chocolate may be thought of as an aphrodisiac; however, the same pleasure chemicals your brain releases when you eat chocolate are the ones you will need for a strong orgasm. If she is already experiencing the pleasure high through her foods, the orgasm she achieves may seem rubbery or less intense.

Massage, music, touching and gentle laughter are all excellent forms of foreplay to enhance a woman's orgasm. The stimulation of touch combined with the mental stimuli and emotional engagement lets the brain know that something special is happening. Laughter helps open up the respiratory system a bit and relaxes the muscles in a natural way so that your erogenous zones are ready for the kind of pulse that is going to make everything tingle and carry her to the release she desire.

12. Orgasms were once prescribed to promote mental health

Throughout the ages sex has been a pivotal and misunderstood part of culture. Depending on the religion, sophistication, and ideology of a culture, the role of orgasm and the sexual organs of women have played an important component in shaping societal habits and values.

The early Celtic and naturalist cultures saw women as empowered beings because of their ability to give birth and worshipped the ability to transmit life through goddess culture and theology. For many of those earth faiths orgasm was seen as a sort of "possession" by the goddess and a form or magic that could protect people and give visions.

When the Roman army conquered the Celtic people, sex was one of the many weapons they used to enslave and shame women in an attempt to replace the power of life giving (by birth) with the power of life taking (by the sword). That shame and the whispered "magic" of orgasm continued on through time.

In the Victorian age, women displaying any number of illnesses (depression, schizophrenia, fatigue, personality disorders, anger management issues, hormonal imbalance) were diagnosed as having "hysteria," a catch-all phrase suggesting problems with a woman's reproductive system (largely still a mystery in the Victorian age) were causing the various ailments.

The theory of hysteria was loosely based on the observation of male physicians that only women seemed to be troubled by many of these issues and since the ability to reproduce is the obvious difference it must be the cause. For women with advanced cases doctors gave them a hysterectomy, but for women with intermittent symptoms doctors prescribed orgasms.

The same observational skills that led physicians to believe only women suffered from depression, insanity or anger also informed them that once a woman has had an orgasm she is pleasant, docile and easy to get along with. Doctors prescribed masturbation or "clinics" where "specialists" would manually masturbate women to orgasm as a way of controlling the hysteria.

Of course, they had no way of knowing the chemicals released during orgasm are the same ones that provide pleasure and muscular release. They just knew many women seemed to get along better with others and seem less edgy when they were having regular orgasms.

In a society where women were subject to a million social and sexual rules like Victorian England, telling someone to go home and masturbate was a big deal. Even more of a change was the idea women should let another man, not her husband, manually stimulate her. However, under the veil of "medical science" women were finally encouraged and allowed to see to their own pleasure.

To make it easier and less socially awkward, a new machine was invented to help women cure their hysteria quickly and easily. That machine was the vibrator. It was less awkward than an appointment with a stranger, and there was no shame because it served a "medical purpose."

Now we understand that having an orgasm won't cure mental health issues or physical diseases. However, if you're a bit on edge or just need a little help smiling through your day, a quick and easy orgasm might be just "what the doctor ordered."

13. (For Her) You cannot get addicted to your vibrator

A prevalent myth that circulates social circles when talk about vibrators comes up is the idea that a woman can become "addicted" to her vibrator. The conversation also crops up in a relationship when a husband or boyfriend doesn't want their partner to use a vibrator for stimulation. Groups that have religious ideas against masturbation have successfully (in some places) petitioned governments to create bans on sex toys, particularly the vibrator, by claiming it is harmful to relationships and the women who use them.

A vibrator isn't a drug, a contributor to sexual delinquency, or unsafe in any way. In fact, far from being a home-wrecker, a vibrator often becomes a marriage saver by ensuring a woman gets sexual satisfaction as part of her relationship. Sexologists frequently recommend vibrators for women who have trouble achieving orgasm through intercourse or manual/oral stimulation. The concentration of stimulation is what many women need to learn to "open the door." There are no studies or indications of any kind that once a woman has orgasms with a vibrator she can only have them that way.

Every touch is different and new touches or sensations are often more delightful and arousing than the same old feeling. So, the way it feels when your partner touches, licks or enters you is going to be entirely different from the way a vibrator is going to feel. Add to the sensation the emotional elements of love, lust or interest and the feelings of being with your partner are going to create healthy satisfaction just as easily as it always has. The vibrator is a tool, not a replacement.

There is no law that says a woman who needs or uses a vibrator to achieve orgasms has to be alone when that happens. Vibrators can be used by a couple during their intercourse or before/after in order to enhance the whole experience. Trusting your lover to use his mouth on your clitoris is one thing, trusting him to hold a moving machine going 300 RPM per second is a much higher level! Many vibrators are designed with remote switches, curves and handles so couples can share and enjoy the vibrations together.

Vibrators come in a variety of shapes and sizes. Because of those 8,000 nerve endings in the clitoris, women are going to do better with indirect stimulation around the clitoral hood or sides of the vulva than applying a direct current right to the clitoris itself.

For hands-free vibration there are small wave vibrators, usually in the shape of a butterfly, that can be strapped around the pelvis which allows them to sit on top of the clitoral hood or be placed over the nether lips to provide an extra charge.

A hand-held, but smaller, alternative is the "Pocket Rocket" (often sold in stores as a hand massager). This small cylinder has a powerful vibration, is tiny enough to conceal in your hand and takes 1 AA battery. The drawback to the pocket rocket is its volume. Having such a powerful little engine in a small plastic case creates a lot of noise.

The vibrator sexologists recommend most for a woman seeking orgasm or for couples wanting to enhance the energy of their love making is the Fukuoku. This tiny vibrator from Japan, originally designed to relieve headaches, fits on the base of a finger (yours or your lover's) and provides focused, pulsing stimulation. The ingenious design lets the vibrator go anywhere a finger might go. The Fukuoku can be found in almost any online sex toy site, in sex shops, and some health and wellness boutiques (you know, in case you have a "headache").

For women who want to add more vaginal stimulation or vibrations to the pelvic floor, a vibrating dildo or egg vibrator placed inside a penis-shaped dildo will certainly do the trick. Woman who are looking for a "full pelvic stimulation" should invest in a "Rabbit" type vibrator (the classic style looked like a bunny but there are many animals now) where a vibrating or swiveling prong (sometimes with a base filled with ball-bearings for extra stimulation) is inserted vaginally and an extension (the bunny ears) stimulate the clitoris as the same time. A vibrating anal plug can be added to the mix to bring even more sensual energy to your brain.

It is important to note, and to reassure your lover, that no amount of silicone, plastic, batteries, wires, ball-bearings or bumps is ever going to take the place of the emotional, personal and relational feelings you get from sex with your partner. Vibrators aren't any more addicting than the spatulas you use to cook or the toothbrush that helps you keep your teeth clean. A vibrator is just another tool in your growing sexual repertoire.

14. The G-Spot isn't really a thing

The vibrators you may not want to spend a lot of money and time on are the so-called "G-Spot" vibrators. These often look like long wands with a curl on the end (frighteningly shaped like a dentist's mirror) and are designed to hit the "G-Spot" in order to produce the elusive G-Spot orgasm.

That would all be wonderful if the G-Spot really existed. However, researchers have long held that the magical G-Spot, and its mythical orgasmic abilities does not follow any kind of consistent, predictable pattern and simply isn't real.

The news comes as a shock to many women who have heard through women's magazines (Cosmo is the number one perpetrator of the myth), sexy shows on late night TV, and vibrator ads that there is an amazing little spot on the front of the vaginal wall at the meeting of the vaginal opening and urethra meet.

This super sensitive spot is supposed to be so connected to vaginal nerves that stimulation or repeated contact can trigger an earth shattering vaginal/clitoral orgasm. Survey says: not so.

Ernst Gräfenberg, a German gynecologist who specialized in studying female ejaculation (also not really a thing) believed he had discovered an area right in front of the urethra that when given firm, pulsing pressure could trigger female ejaculation and strong orgasms. This area was eventually named after him, and reduced to the nickname "the G-Spot."

However, during the rest of his research and practice, other researchers considered his findings to be unsubstantiated and most of his research was conducted through anecdotal evidence of participants in the studies. Some scientists think the area is just the Skene's gland – a sort of female version of the prostate – and has no unique or distinct sexual characteristic whatsoever.

Some women (a large number of which were taught to believe in the G-Spot) do report extra sensitivity and arousal if that area is stimulated. However, every woman is different and what might be an erogenous zone in one woman is not necessarily a trigger for another. For every woman who claims the G-Spot gives her the best orgasms ever, there are four other women who are frustrated or feel badly because they can't find "the spot" or it just doesn't do anything for them.

The answer to the G-Spot controversy in terms of orgasm is very simple. If you can't find it, stop looking for it. It probably isn't going to help you. If there is a pleasure spot in her vaginal channel that makes her feel great – by all means stimulate it and enjoy it. Don't get hung up on the myths of what the female body is "supposed to be." Learn to explore and enjoy her own body, no matter where the pleasure comes from.

15. (For Her) Fantasy is required

The G-Spot may not exist for every woman everywhere, but there is one thing that is a constant in women's ability to achieve orgasm – the presence of fantasy or brain engagement. Since the 1950's when research into women's sexual responses was in its infancy, one thing has been proven in every kind of study – quantitative, qualitative and anecdotal.

Women have to be actively engaged in a sexual thought for orgasms to occur. You can't lay there and think about the grocery list and expect to experience the bliss of release. The brain must be actively imagining or thinking about sexuality in order to release the right reflex at the best time.

For women who are engaging in self-sexuality, fantasizing about being involved in a sex act is usually the key to building sufficient tense and biomedical release. Remember, your brain can't really see. So if it is feeling stimulation coupled with the fantasy of you making love to George Clooney, your brain will believe you really are making love to George Clooney and release the sexual chemicals your body requires for orgasms.

If you are trying to grow closer to your spouse or lover, however, it would be better to fantasize about being with him, or at least running through your mind feelings and ideas about what you are sexually doing with him. This not only encourages your brain to understand sex is happening, but will tie the thoughts of pleasure and release to your spouse, creating a mental association between him and pleasure.

If you aren't thinking sexual thoughts (real or imagined) your brain may interpret the stimuli as pain, or a bug on your skin and release a lot of adrenaline to make you restless or release some endorphins to deal with pain, but the combination required for sexual release will not occur.

One of the reasons so many religions have been against masturbation is the presence of what they consider to be "lustful fantasies" as a key element in the science of orgasm. However, masturbation and release of sexual tension is a very natural, healthy thing to do. People who try to repress those natural urges and fight off sexual thoughts, often find themselves experiencing sex dreams as their subconscious mind seeks to stimulate the brain into releasing the hormones. In men, that creates nocturnal emissions. In women, they may wake us wet from arousal but rarely achieve orgasm in their sleep.

While it takes a lot of stimulation, pleasure and pulsing for your body to have an orgasm, you can't forget your mind. You must be engaged mentally in order for your orgasm to occur. In the words of Homer Simpson, "think sexy thoughts!"

16. (For Her) The best way to have an orgasm is to stop trying to have an orgasm

Orgasms are like cats. The more you want them to come to you, the farther away they tend to stay. Due to the effect of psychological stress on the brain, worrying about your relationship or trying to have an orgasm actually decreases the chances you will find that sweet release. The best state for a mind/body to be in for sexual satisfaction is a relaxed state.

The primary question that inhibits the brain's ability to achieve release is, "why are you trying so hard to have an orgasm?" If a relationship is stalling, sexually or personally, many women think increasing the amount of sexual pleasure will help ease tension or reaffirm their devotion to their partner. However, when the desire for orgasm is coupled with feelings about strain or danger to the relationship the brain tends to sort out the sexual urges and focus on the concern instead. This limits the sexual imagery in the brain and makes it hard to concentrate on pleasure.

The same effect can also occur if you are worried about your health or sexual prowess and are attempting to have an orgasm because you haven't had one, or feel somehow "less than" because of your rate of orgasmic response. Whether self-pressure, social pressure or spousal pressure – that kind of tension is retroactive to achieving the desired sexual plateau.

In response to stress the brain releases cortisol, one of the brain's pain relievers, instead of the endorphins that create pleasure. When cortisol is released the best feeling a woman can achieve is numbness. Cortisol has an important place in our brain's catalogue of survival hormones, but long-term releasing of cortisol (due to stress, sleep deprivation, worry or depression) causes serious side effects, including increased blood sugar, an overage of calcium, increased heart rate and decreased response reflexes. Cortisol is the reason stress causes heart attack and stroke. Imagine what it's doing to your sex life.

Fortunately, some of the best types of foreplay are also known as cortisol reducers. Soft music has been proven to reduce cortisol levels through relaxing and enveloping the mind with signals telling the brain to increase feeling, not decrease it. Touch is another good cortisol reducer along with laughter. Interestingly, studies show dancing reduces cortisol and increases the amount of adrenaline leading to the perfect scenario for enhanced sexual pleasure.

The next time you want an evening to end with a beautiful orgasm, forget about that. Go dancing, turn on soft music, have a massage and laugh with your lover. By the time you are involved in your sexual expression your brain will be fully engaged and ready to empower the very feelings you are seeking. As an added bonus, the effect of the cortisol reducing stress busters also creates strong feelings and good memories with your lover. You'll not only be having a great time but the disconnect you were fearing will be alleviated as well.

17. (For Her) The best time to have an orgasm is at the beginning of sex

It has long been a topic of joking conversations and an envious revelation that women are capable of multiple orgasms in a small amount of time. But, the female brain, much like the male brain, needs some kind of respite and only has so many muscle control chemicals to release at any given time. So, the first orgasm is always going to be the stronger one, marked by increased release. However, the second one is easier to achieve (due to the fact the brain has already produced the pleasure chemicals for use) and usually has a different emotional and personal feel to it.

Even if a woman is not seeking two orgasms, having one before intercourse begins will make intercourse more pleasurable and increase the likelihood of an orgasm more focused on the pelvic floor if the second one occurs.

Women who sometimes experience pain during intercourse are encouraged to have an orgasm before sexual entry. Having your lover give you an orgasm though oral or manual stimulation dramatically increases the amount of vaginal lubrication and amount of blood flow to your pelvic area. Your vaginal channel will already be swelling and prepared for sexual intercourse and your brain will be locked in and ready to continue providing necessary support. When your body is more prepared, the pain and stretching of intercourse is reduced and the experience is more pleasurable all around.

If your partner does not choose to give you an orgasm first, the next best time to have one is after he climaxes. The act of intercourse itself will stimulate the clitoris and send nerve signals up to the brain. However, many women get lost in the actions of their partner or own physical disconnect and are unable to experience the thoughts necessary to promote an orgasmic response. The best thing to do in that case is to wait until your partner is finished and has ejaculated.

Begin to do kegel-like exercises and continue moving your hips and pelvic area as if intercourse is still going on. Keep your mind engaged, thinking about the sexual moment with him. Take his hand and place it where you want it or ask him to use his mouth to give you increased impulses (if he balks at oral sex after his ejaculation, remind him it is just a simple body fluid and you taste it all the time). If your partner is falling asleep or is just not willing/able to stimulate you – masturbate while continuing the scenario in your mind until you achieve release.

Mutual orgasm is commonly held up as the sort of "holy grail" of sexuality. However, from a physical and psychosexual standpoint, it's not that great. For one thing, when you are both engaged in orgasm at the same time, a woman's inclination is usually to cater to his pleasure and she can't concentrate or feel as much of her own pleasure occurring. Add to that the reality the brain is already overloaded with your demands and is now being asked to be conscious of another person's pleasure and impulses. It tends to lead to mental/physical shut down. A more organic "feel it when I feel it" approach to orgasm is a much better choice.

18. Position matters

Although there are about 12 prime sexual positions and at least 100 slight variations of each, the average couple has a sexual repertoire of about four positions, one of which is the good old standard missionary position. That's a shame because the position of your bodies during intercourse can help or hinder a number of components including lubrication, pregnancy, depth and orgasm. If she is not experiencing orgasms during intercourse, be a little adventurous and give some other positions a try.

Great positions for orgasm usually include placing each body in such a way the vaginal area, pelvic floor and the clitoral area all receive stimulation from the natural movements or thrusts of sex. While some may sound a little physically awkward at first, experiment with them and encourage your partner to experience some of the joy, laughter, and newness that comes along with doing something different.

Remember, if you do what you have always done, you'll just keep on getting what you've always gotten.

Good positions for orgasm include:

- **Fold in half**: Don't worry, it's not as extreme as it sounds. The woman lies on her back, with a pillow under her butt to raise it to a better angle. Lifting her legs (with a partner's help if necessary) she brings them back toward her shoulders – as if she is folding in half. After her partner inserts his penis, she can bring her legs back down to rest on his shoulders. This gives the penetration a lot of depth, and the elevation of hips allows his body to pulse against the clitoral hood.

- **Facedown on the bed**: When most people think of "doggy style" they are imagining rear-entry vaginal sex with a woman bent over the bed (or table, desk, arm of a chair) or on all fours. There's a better way. Have the woman lie face down on top of the bed and lift her butt just slightly so her partner can gain entry. This employs good body mechanics with the spine, is not tiring for her legs and as he is thrusting in her vaginally, she can grind her clitoris against the bed to create a critical mass of stimulation.

- **Reverse Cowgirl**: One of the more popular "woman on top" positions, reverse cowgirl offers the ability not only to control the depth and angle of the thrust but also leaves the clitoral area easy to access for manual self-stimulation. In reverse cowgirl the man lies on the bed and the woman mounts his penis, facing away from him. Using her hip/thigh muscles she provides the motion, while at the same time she can reach down and stimulate her clitoris.

- **The Lap Dance:** Why not bring the whole body into the mix? Instead of "woman on top," the lap dance is actually "both on top" which allows for a myriad of things to happen all at the same time. The man sits up (in a chair or on a bed against the headboard) and the woman straddles his penis, facing him as she "sits on his lap". This is a much less athletic position than reverse cowgirl. Instead of just going up and down, she can move side-to-side, sway, and jolt her hips. His waist is pressed against her clitoris giving it plenty of stimulation as she moves, and the position allows him access to her breasts, or mouth or anything he wants to kiss. The increase in intimacy empowers the couple to experience stronger sensations throughout intercourse.

- **The Spoon**: Emotional intimacy, security and connection are all part of having an orgasm during intercourse and no position offers that better than the spoon. The woman lies on her side and her partner scoots right up against her back, inserting himself in her vaginally from behind. The downside to spooning during intercourse is that it doesn't allow for deep penetration which is a minus if you want to make babies. However, the plus is that the position holds the penis against the front of the vaginal wall which is great for orgasm. Instead of thrusting in and out, the man should keep his position in relatively the same place and move his hips allowing him to slowly, rhythmically stimulate the vaginal wall. He can reach around and rub her clitoris while enveloping her body in warmth and good feelings. The nice part about the spoon is that after the orgasm has rocked both your worlds, you two are in the perfect position to go to sleep.

Any position that allows for both vaginal and clitoral stimulation is going to make having an orgasm easier. So saddle up, or spoon on down and give these a try.

19. There is no magical pill for orgasm

The power of sex and the allure of complete sexual satisfaction are ideas humans are willing to pursue no matter how odd or unproven the tactics may be. From our earliest days, men and women have been searching for pills, roots, solutions and methods to ensure arousal. It is such a primal draw for us that most of the aphrodisiac myths we believe about food, salves, and spells were actually created by merchants. Sellers knew getting people to believe the item can increase pleasure and lead to orgasm would increase the market share. Science tells a different story.

In orgasm there are two important chemicals, serotonin and dopamine. Any food or process that causes the brain to release those chemicals is considered a help in terms of arousal and good feelings. However, they are not enough to trigger the reflex women need to feel in order to experience orgasm.

Food aphrodisiacs sound like a good plan until you really dig into their stories and recognize the truth inside them. In the case of avocados, story is all there is to find. Avocados have been considered an aphrodisiac because of the shape of the fruit itself. Avocados were first used by the Aztecs as a sexual enhancement food. They named it "ahuacatl", which means "testicle". That's the only sexual claim avocados have. They look like testicles.

Some foods make, at least initially, a more compelling case. Chocolate, particularly dark chocolate, releases dopamine into the system which makes a person relax and feel pleasurable. Remember, your brain only has so much dopamine on tap. If you release it all eating vast amounts of chocolate you are more likely to end up feeling sleepy and satisfied, not sexy and wanting. Oysters have zinc which increases the rate of blood flow – that causes arousal. But, in order to get the kind of blood flow that would actually empower your body for an orgasm, you would have to eat a bathtub full.

Age-old roots and herbs also don't provide any scientifically viable effects. Pheromone stimulation, the idea that certain primal, sexual scents our bodies send out can lead to increased sexual interest, has also not been proven in scientific study. Rose petals, gingerbread and musk may do some good if the smell relaxes a person or gives them pleasant memories. But, none of those smells, oils or infusions are going to make a difference in the long run.

Orgasm is best achieved through a loving, intimate connection that leads to proper stimulation of the right nerve endings and a brain understanding the signals and getting things done. All the other ideas are just tastes and fantasy from days gone by.

20. Orgasm is not a sign of sexual experience or maturity

The myth used to be that the quicker she had an orgasm the more sexually mature or experienced she was. Like many myths, this idea is rooted in a male dominated culture promoting the idea that a woman who experiences and expresses sexual pleasure is promiscuous or perverted in some fashion. The inability of women to experience sexual release was connected to youth, virginity and purity.

In reality, orgasm is a healthy reflex that can occur in any woman at any time. Having an orgasm quickly doesn't make her a deviant and having one that builds over the course of your sexual experience doesn't mean she is pure and faithful. Orgasm depends on the body and brain of the individual at the moment in question. There is no vice or virtue shown by a woman's speed, strength, length or response to orgasm.

21 Orgasm has a purpose

Biological anthropologists and medical historians are often involved in the hunt for why our bodies are made the way they are and how it affects our long-term health and survival as a species. The clitoris has long been a subject of research in both the anatomical and ethical disciplines. This small part of the body so full of nerve endings seems to exist solely for pleasure. It doesn't help in procreation and doesn't make sex more possible or viable.

Scientists have now turned their understandings of orgasm away from the search for meaning in the body parts themselves, and toward an understanding of the process of orgasm. One of the primary chemicals released by the brain during orgasm is oxytocin. Not only does it enhance sexual experiences but it is also a factor in psychological pair bonding, social recognition, desire, and contentment. In short, this brain chemical makes people love one another.

Anthropologists tend to believe that orgasm serves a great role in survival by creating bond-pairing and trust between people. The shared experiences associated with orgasm, an intensely intimate act, create trust between people which allows us to stay together, build stronger relationships and family units, and solidify commitment with our partners. Orgasms don't just make sex great; they make society stronger and survival inevitable.

No matter how much we know about orgasms – their cause, their effects, their history and their future – we will never know all we need to know about this illusive reflex. As scientists, scholars, sexologists and everyday people continue to discover – orgasm is an unraveling miracle with more secrets, stories and power than we will ever understand.

Part II: 27 Techniques to Give Her Mind Blowing Pleasure

From the fact that major receptors for sexual pleasure are deeply hidden under folds of skin, to the reality that the most important sexual organ, the brain, requires emotional connection as well as physical stimulation, women are outlandishly sexually complex. Their orgasms can range in intensity from barely noticeable to earth shattering with a host of sensations in between.

In order to give the woman of your dreams orgasms on a consistent basis (or even just one really unforgettably expressive one) there are techniques you will need to employ.

Here are 27 techniques you can use to ensure your partner has an immensely pleasurable climax. The techniques are broken up into 3 categories: **Foreplay**, **Techniques**, and **Positions**. You don't have to do all of them all at once, but give these tips a try and you'll find her rocking and rolling in your arms in no time.

Foreplay

1. Take Your Time

Not only do women and men have different psychological ideas involving the requirements for the body to achieve orgasm, researches show they also have different physiological needs. Not only do they think differently about sex, their bodies process things differently.

Men achieve orgasm much more quickly and easily than women do. This fact was underscored by research at the Kinsey Institute for Research in Sex, Gender and Reproduction that revealed a woman's body must experience arousal and stimulation for at least 20 minutes before she can have an orgasm.

Don't be afraid. That doesn't mean you have to have intercourse or provide cunnilingus for 20 solid minutes. What it does mean is that you need to engage in a lot of pre-intercourse touching, kissing, and foreplay before switching over to the main event.

Take your time. Don't rush the sexual experience. Make sure you have enough time for foreplay, intercourse and afterglow. Studies also show that if you stop stimulation or touching immediately after her orgasm, it can actually prolong the amount of time it takes for her to have one in the future because her mind will associate climax with the end of the affection and hold off as long as possible.

So, make sure nothing is rushed and your sexual event proceeds at a steady, erotic pace.

2. Start from Afar

In any other part of life waiting for something can be an aggravating and destructive sensation. It can cause you to act impatiently and ruin your mood. When it comes to giving your lover the orgasm of a lifetime, however, anticipation is a very good thing.

Make plans for a big night out and special session of lovemaking. Don't just wait for the moment to arrive. Start early that morning with a note or call before work. Send her text messages throughout the day – some nice and some naughty – that excite her about the evening to come.

A woman wants to feel appreciated and needs to be affirmed about the sexiness and desirability of her body. Start her morning with a note or text that reads, "Can't wait to get my hands on you tonight." If you write it out as a note, be creative and leave a thumb print or draw a hand on the note.

As the day continues, keep upping the ante by sending comments such as "Heard some classic rock music at lunch today. I'm ready to rock with you tonight." Don't be gross, graphic or unnecessarily explicit. The point is to peak her interest and make her feel excited.

You aren't sexting her or trying to get her off over the phone. Keep it light, corny and fun. By the time you two get together, she'll already be interested in everything you want to do, because she's been thinking about it all day too.

3. Play the Brain Game

If you want to get a woman interested in you, tickle her funny bone. If you want a woman to agree to have sex with you, touch her heart. And, if you want a woman to have an amazing orgasm you're going to have to reach for nothing less than her mind.

The brain is the most important and active sexual organ. Not only does it regulate the muscle tension and endorphin release that causes climax, it must also be assured there is a real, visceral and emotional connection before it will produce the biomedical chemicals necessary for orgasm to occur.

For a man to climax, his brain just needs to think, "Wow, this feels good." For a woman to climax she needs to think, "Wow, this feels good because he really cares about me and wants me to know that he is trying to give me pleasure so we can continue to build a relationship together."

When you think about it, that's a lot of responsibility to place on your body. So, don't wait until you are in the act of lovemaking to convey that feeling. Use your words. Talk to your partner and assure her of your care, love and desire for her to experience pleasure.

Don't wait for her to figure those things out on her own. Shower her with affection and let her know up front you want her to have the best sexual experience possible because of the way you feel about her. A few good words in the beginning can save you from a lot of frustration at the end.

4. Wine to Water

It is not uncommon for a woman to have a drink or two to unwind and prepare for sexual intercourse. In fact, many sexually inexperienced women will purposely drink wine with the hopes it will help them through the nervousness of their early sexual experiences.

While it is true that a small amount of alcohol can lower your partner's inhibitions and loosen her up to be more comfortable with sexuality, you always want to make sure you know what her limit is and stop before she gets to it.

In small doses alcohol may make a partner livelier, however, alcohol is a depressant and a numbing agent. The more alcohol she has in her system the more likely she is to either fall asleep, lose focus, or fail to have an orgasm because of the buzzy-numbing effect going on in her head.

Start out with a bottle of wine or a mixed drink but switch to water before the night is through. A good rule of thumb is wait one hour per every drink with a 3 drink maximum (that, of course, depends on the drink. 3 glasses of wine is not the same as 3 Long Island Ice Teas).

If she has wine with dinner, talk and take your time with foreplay until an hour has passed. Talk to her and keep an eye on her response. If she is too drunk to follow what you are saying, she's too drunk to have an orgasm.

5. Wild Whispers

One great way to connect to her head and her lower regions all at the same time is whisper in her ear. In terms of body mechanics, the ears and the area around them are highly erogenous zones. Ears experience sensual pleasure and translate it into sexual impulses.

Often the feel of your breath against her ear will seem to send a sensation directly to her moistening cleft. Not only will a whisper cause a nearly immediate bodily reaction, but the words you say can also go a long way to creating an intimate connection as well.

Some women like to hear "sweet nothings" – nice little sayings and phrases about how beautiful she is, how much you desire or feelings you have for her. Other women are attracted to something a little raunchier – talk about what you want to do to her that is more graphic and "dirty."

If you aren't sure whether your love likes it "naughty or nice" go with the "nice." It is easier to take nice phrases and make them rougher than to take back a rough phrase that is offensive. Either way, make sure your breath doesn't smell (the ears are awfully close to the nose) and that you have sucked all the spit from the front of your mouth and lips. Having someone spit in your ear is not sexy.

Don't know what to say? Check out my book: "131 Dirty Talk Examples: Learn How To Talk Dirty with These Simple Phrases That Drive Your Lover Wild & Beg You For Sex Tonight" - available at all major book retailers.

6. Kiss Her Cares Away

Since you have almost 20 minutes before your lover can even think about having an orgasm, why not spend about 5 of those minutes kissing?

Making out, particularly kissing on the lips, is a tremendous turn-on for women. The intimate connection helps her brain establish the kind of emotional stronghold that will allow her to reach a climax and it shows her you are being a considerate lover by spending time on something she likes as part of your sexual experience.

Scientifically, kissing has a lot of benefits. Studies show the act of kissing actually lowers cortisol (a brain chemical that comes from stress) in the system. Kissing will help relax your lover (without the numbing side effects of wine) and put her in a happier state of being.

A relaxed mind that isn't distracted by the issues and worries of the day is much more likely to connect quickly and experience stronger sensations of arousal. Spending time kissing also shows your lover that sex may be your goal, but connection is really what you're all about. This thought will definitely encourage her to lower her barriers. Soon she will be rocking underneath you with wild abandon.

7. Copious Compliments

In a world full of media, advertisements, and negative people almost all women emerge from adolescence with a plate full of low self-esteem and body issues. Women worry about their size, shape, the color of their areola, their pubic hair, their smell, and more. Even when you've been very upfront about the fact you find your partner desirable the slightest thing can cause her brain to go into overdrive.

It is difficult for her to let go and enjoy the pleasure of your tongue running over her most sensitive places if all she can think about is, "I hope my hair isn't a turn-off" or "I hope he doesn't notice the mole on my stomach." It's probable she will never voice those fears out loud, and she doesn't want to have a conversation about them. But, they're there.

The way to combat that level of insecurity is to compliment her, sincerely, a lot. Take time to say small things like, "I love your breasts" while you are kissing them or when you lean down to provide oral pleasure tell her you love doing that for her and you love her body.

Watch out for backhanded compliments like, "you have such a great butt for someone your age." That will backfire in a hurry and she will shut down completely. You'll be working yourself into exhaustion on her lower half while all her head is doing is planning her entry into the old folk's home. Straightforward, nice compliments are the way to go.

Techniques

8. Who's On First

Obviously a big part of your desire to give your partner the ultimate sexual pleasure has to do with your care and concern for her. However, it is also true that you want to have a good sexual experience as well. Sex is, after all, a mutually beneficial experience.

The best thing to do in order to create an amazing sexual event for yourself is to put her first. Focus on the things she likes – whether it is kissing, touching, naughty talk, spanking, holding, or licking. Enticing her body and sensual needs will put her in a better position to be able to meet your needs as well.

Evidence is overwhelming that men think far more about sex and think more often about sex than women. The old saying, "men only want one thing" may have some basis in truth. However, equally true is the saying, "women want to be that one thing." Being the initiator and putting her needs and desires first will help her understand she is the one you want.

Don't wait for her to reach down and unzip your pants. Reach out to her and touch her first. Encourage her to experience arousal then channel it back to your own needs. Don't be overly aggressive (women don't like to feel like a potato chip bag you just grab and use for your satisfaction), but do be assertive and initiate sexual expression.

9. Shoot for Two

This wouldn't be a guide about orgasms if it didn't mention at least a couple of times that women have a great advantage when it comes to pleasure. Women can have multiple orgasms. It may take a bit of effort to get her body and brain on the track toward climax, but when it arrives a woman can achieve release again and again.

For men, once ejaculation has occurred the sexual event is over – at least for a half-hour or so. For women, the first orgasm can be just a warm up to a hotter release yet-to-come. With that in mind, don't be stingy with her orgasms. Start her off with one, and then see to your own pleasure.

Research proves that strong vaginal orgasms are more likely to happen after she has already experienced a smaller climax. The best method of assuring a memorable moment is to see to her pleasure first and use your hand or mouth to stimulate her into a first orgasm. That experience will increase her heart rate, lubrication level, and brain chemistry so her body will be poised and ready for the second, mind-blowing release.

It is not recommended for you to use a vibrator for her first orgasm. The speed and strength of the vibrations will make her come quickly but, it can also create over-stimulation or a numbing experience that makes it harder for the second one to be felt as strongly.

Remember, in women an orgasm isn't necessarily the end of the event; it might just be the beginning.

10. Save the Best for Last

An athlete in any sport will tell you that you never bring your "A" game to practice or warm up. You save it for when the real game actually begins. The same is true for sex. Don't get so excited about giving her that first orgasm that you rush the beginning process and head straight to her mound for oral stimulation. Save it for later.

Men's sexual feelings are generally focused in the genital/pelvic area. However, women's sexual arousal encompasses more of her full body. Her breasts, neck, back, hips and even thighs all generate sexual sensations that trigger lubrication and prepare her for climax. If you kiss her a few minutes then rush straight to her clitoral area to begin oral sex you are likely to shut her down.

A woman's clitoris has more nerve endings than any other part of the human body. It is an extremely sensitive area. If she is not mentally and physically ready for oral stimulation, your quick action is more likely to over-stimulate her and cause the process to stop. Instead of running her hand through your hair as you tongue her, she will be pushing your head back and moving away.

Start with her head and neck and slowly kiss your way down to her vaginal area. Spend time lightly touching and rubbing her mound. Then when she is warmed up and receptive, move in and begin slowly licking and nurturing her clit. Oral sex is not the start line. It's the point mid-race when you make a break and head toward the finish.

11. Never Try Dry

For men one of the best sensations in sex is the heat that comes from the friction of the penis rubbing against the walls of the vagina. Women enjoy that sensation as well. However, that channel happens to be a sensitive mucosal tissue inside her body. Without proper lubrication the experience turns from being sexy and pleasurable to being raw, stinging and unpleasant.

A well- oiled machine is sexy. Sandpaper is not. Always make sure to use enough lubrication to ensure the ability to slide in and out of her body easily. There will still be plenty of heat and friction as her body will form to your penis and grasp it when her pleasure increases.

It is true that women self-lubricate and men generate a certain amount of pre-cum in order to help the process along. However, neither women nor men make enough natural lubricant for the process to be completely comfortable or create the kind of stimulation that results in orgasm.

Make sure you not only use lube when you insert your penis into her, but also put a little bit on your fingers if you are going to finger her first (recommended to get her inner core ready to receive you). Nothing stops arousal for a woman like a bone dry finger prying into her soft, fleshy vaginal channel.

Don't shy away from a lot of lube. Sex is wet. Sex is messy. That's where all the magic happens.

12. Play in the Zone

Women's magazines and popular sex books spend the majority of their informational space talking about the G-spot, that magical button inconveniently hidden inside a woman's vagina that makes her climax like a plug has been put in a socket and 50,000 volts are going through her body.

Unfortunately, as mentioned, the mythical G-spot is just that. Mostly, a myth. Women DO have sensitive places in their vaginal wall or on the pelvic floor that increase their sensation. But, it is not "one spot," it is not in the same place in all women, and it does not always have the same result.

A better way of creating a strong orgasm in your partner is to understand the G-spot as a "zone", not a "spot." Spend time with your fingers or penis during foreplay or the beginning of intercourse touching different areas and pushing at different angles (changing sexual positions will give you more knowledge of how her body works and where her arousal zone might be) so you can discover what really makes her feel good. That's the fun part of a sexual relationship – the voyage of discovery and experience.

If you approach every woman thinking, "Your G-spot is at the forward top of your vaginal wall and when I stimulate it you're going to explode with pleasure," you are going to be setting yourself and your lover up for a big disappointment.

Take your time, work with her, and play around. When you find it – you'll know it.

13. Multitask

The basic biology of orgasm for women is that stimulation causes the tissue and muscles of their pelvic area to become so constricted and tight (almost like a cramp) that they need release. Once a woman's body crosses the threshold of what it can endure the brain kicks in to provide a series of chemicals that release all the muscles at once, providing uncontrollable waves of pleasurable feelings.

In order to create the ultimate orgasm, you want to make sure to stimulate as many of those muscle groups as possible. The more areas she has constricted, the stronger the orgasm will be as she releases.

Involve your partner's whole body in her orgasm. While you are tightening and delighting the pelvic floor with your thrusts, reach up (or reach around) and use your hands to stimulate her clitoris, or encourage her to rub her own clitoris while you use your hands to knead her breasts or buttocks. Use your mouth to tantalize her nipples. Any part of her that you can touch, lick, bite or suck – use it to bring her entire body on board for the climax of her life.

14. Look Her in the Eye

Sexual intercourse is not like grocery shopping where you go down the list checking each thing off until you finally end up at the check-out counter. It isn't like: emotional connection? Check. Kissing? Check. Oral? Check. Penetration? Check. Liftoff!!! It is more like a running track where you go by the same milestones over and over – each lap coming with a little more heavy breathing, deeper meaning and then you cross the finish line (and run a little ways farther to keep everything in good working order). So, once you've penetrated your partner, don't think the emotional connection part is over for the night. Keep doing it.

Since the middle of intercourse is not a great time to start a conversation about how amazing your partner is, the best way to keep that connection is to look at her. Eyes are the windows of the soul and when you two make a visual connection with one another during the course of your passion, everything will lock into place.

One of the top pieces of advice sex educators give women who want to learn how to give a good blow job is to make eye contact.

The same holds true for you guys. If you are having sex in a position where you can't see her face (reverse cowgirl, doggy style, etc.) then make sure to look at her in the afterglow.

Afterglow isn't about the sex you just had. It's about the sex you're going to have next. Keep that connection strong.

15. Rock Concert

One of the most important phrases a man can hear about how to be an incredible lover is this: rock, don't pound.

After penetration men too often focus on thrusting or make the mistake of thinking "harder/faster" is the best way to bring a woman to orgasm. Slapping against her and pounding yourself home may seem good in porn movies and erotica, but in reality it doesn't work out that well.

The force of hard thrusting jars the lower back, rubs the vaginal channel raw and, depending on the length of your penis, smacks up against the cervix (intensely painful). You know all those guys you hear say, "My wife says sex is painful." as they look sadly at the ground? It's because they are pounding.

Once you enter your lover rock your hips, bringing her body along with you. Move in a fluid rocking motion back and forth, not exiting her body and re-entering and not slamming into her mound. Rocking allows you to move together.

If your lover wants to increase speed or friction she can move with your rhythm, pushing down as you rock into her. This makes sex a joint venture and assures that she is not feeling any discomfort. In order to stun her with a powerful climax remember the adage: "Smooth, fluid motion makes the waves rock the ocean."

16. Waiting is the Hardest Part

Few people receive quality sex education classes or learn from certified sex educators about the best ways to have sex. Most people learn about it by doing it. Many women also adopt sexual attitudes from their mothers, religious leaders, or media.

Culturally, women learn to focus on the needs of men, and wait for men to both initiate and guide intercourse. That becomes a problem when it is time for women to experience a sense of sexual satisfaction.

Once the man ejaculates, women tend to shut down, thinking everything is done. If she hasn't achieved climax it will leave her frustrated and over time she will communicate she isn't satisfied with her sex life.

In order to be a giving lover she appreciates for getting her off, instead of just a sexmate who "comes and goes," it is important you last long enough for her to have an orgasm first.

If you are having intercourse and you feel yourself rising to climax, try to put your mind elsewhere or use as much restraint as you can to keep going. Keep an eye on your partner, if she is close to climaxing too, tell her you are getting ready to come so she can bear down with her hips or stimulate her clitoris to bring her to an even place so you can orgasm together.

After all the foreplay and sensuality you've experienced, you may not be able to hold out very long. If you ejaculate soon after penetration your best course of action would be to masturbate prior to being with your partner so you are working on your second orgasm and will be less likely to ejaculate quickly.

If you want to give her really good orgasms and encourage her sexual participation and satisfaction, wait for her.

17. The 90 Second Window

Stimulation is necessary and connection is important but, when trying to give your partner a heart pounding, body trembling orgasm - timing is everything. Prior to orgasm all women enter what is known as the 90 second window. It's that minute and a half before she climaxes and it is the "make or break" time for the event. Learn to read the signs of the 90 second window so you know exactly when she enters that moment.

How can you tell when a woman is about to climax? There are a number of visual and auditory clues. A woman's back will arch upward and she will usually press her head backwards or down. Her hands may begin to grasp or clamp shut and she will likely close her eyes.

Inside her, you should be able to feel her vaginal walls gripping your penis or rippling along the sides of your shaft. Her hips will move upward and the pelvic floor will rise and tighten. You will also hear a change in her breathing pattern as her heart rate speeds up making her breath come out in ragged bursts.

Women are less likely to be able to tell you when they are about to release because even their jaws lock on occasion. When her whole body begins to curl up and she is breathing more loudly than your background music, you'll know you're in the 90 second window.

18. Steady as She Blows

There are a lot of times to try new tricks and change up what you're doing for effect. During the 90 second window is not that time. No matter what you are doing, whether you are giving her cunnilingus or rocking with a slow and steady rhythm as your penis rubs against her arousal zone, do not stop and do not change.

When a woman enters the 90 second window her body moves to "auto-pilot" and her brain is now running the show and ramping up to release all the tight muscles at once. When you change speed, pressure or sensation during that time it stops the brain for a second as it incorporates the new sensation into the mix. At best you will prolong her wait to orgasm and at worst her brain may completely shut her system down and stop the orgasm right before its time, leaving her tense and frustrated.

The thing you want to do when you notice she is in the 90 second window is pay close attention to whatever you are doing and try to keep your pace and sensation as steady as possible. Once she is that close to the cliff, she doesn't need anything new or extra. Your good lovin' has brought her all the way to the top, let her body take her over the edge. Chances are, if you are close to climax as well, her initial spasms will pull you over the edge with her.

19. Luscious Lips

Men tend to think of the clitoris as that amazing little button which sits under the clitoral hood for the purpose of bringing women to climax. It is true that the clitoris seems to serve no other purpose in the female body but provide sexual pleasure. That little area is home to 8,000 nerve endings.

One thing you may not realize is that the clitoris is not really a button. Underneath the clitoral hood the clitoris has a tendril coming from each side (full of nerve fibers) that extend down the vaginal lips like two little arms. Impulses on the vaginal lips travel up those tendrils directly to the clitoris itself and then straight to the brain. So, when you're down there making sure her clit gets lots of attention, don't forget the lips.

A good technique during oral sex is to start by licking and sucking each lip gently to get her juices flowing and awaken the clitoris to prepare for your arrival. Because it is so super sensitive the clitoris cannot sustain a lot of sudden, sharp or direct contact.

The clit is a shy friend you have to coax from out behind her skirt. Paying attention to the vaginal lips will make that process easier so your stimulation is pleasant and not overbearing. If you are using your hand to arouse your partner, make sure to tweak and rubs the lips as well.

20. Light as a Feather

Direct stimulation of the clitoris is never a good idea. Too much sensation of any area causes the brain to read the signals as "pain" instead of "pleasure" and she will react by pulling away from you. Triggering your lover's "fight or flight" reflex is not a good way to bring her to orgasm.

Approach the area slowly, stroking and giving sensual touch to her vulva, vaginal lips and the top of her mound. This will let her tolerance to the sensation build up naturally and she will welcome more of it.

One advanced technique to bring her to a quick orgasm manually is to lightly rub the sides of the clitoral hood with the tips of your fingers. Start by touching and rubbing her vaginal lips, then you will be able to notice the clitoris rising underneath the clitoral hood. Run your finger back and forth lightly on one side of the clitoral hood. The vibration of the area will make her so sensitive she will swear she can feel the ridges of your fingertips.

If she responds positively to the teasing, light touch, use two fingers and gently rub back and forth on both sides of the clitoral hood. She will be convulsing with pleasure in no time. Because that first orgasm was a clitoral climax, her body will now be ready for penetration and build towards a second, more powerful release.

21. Plug In

Sexual research shows almost all women can achieve orgasm through masturbation and many of them use vibrators or sex toys to help in that process. The intense stimulation of a vibrator or the sensation of using a dildo or butt plug can bring more of a woman's body into the orgasmic process and create a stronger climax.

Don't let her have all that fun alone. Bring the toys into your sex practices as well. The vibrator is not going to replace you. It is going to work with you to help your partner enjoy the most satisfying experience possible.

Encourage your lover to use a butterfly or clitoral vibrator during intercourse so you can stimulate both erogenous zones at the same time. You can even get a remote control vibrator that will allow you to start/stop/change the sensation she feels while you are penetrating her.

If you have ejaculated but she has not had an orgasm yet, withdraw your penis and use a dildo or vibrator to continue stimulation until she completes her release. If it takes her a very long time to climax with cunnilingus, insert a butt plug or anal-safe dildo that you can pull and push in her to add a new or full sensation that creates more muscle tension and stronger orgasms.

Even women with capable, caring lovers use vibrators as part of their sexual repertoire. Make them part of yours too.

Positions

22. Go Against the Grain

No one likes to hear, "you're doing it wrong." But, chances are – when it comes to giving your partner oral sex – you're doing it wrong. Or, at least in the wrong position. Most men position their head in front of the woman's vulva and lick in an up and down fashion, going with the grain so-to-speak.

As cunnilingus continues the male partner may dip his tongue into the vaginal opening or run it up and lick or suck around the clitoral hood. While that is a pleasurable feeling, and no woman is going to complain about a man who wants to give her oral pleasure, the truth is, there is a better way.

Position yourself perpendicular to your partner. So, on a clock if she is lying at 12 – 6, you would be lying at 9 to 3 (or 3 to 9 depending on which side of the bed or couch she is on). Lick across her vulva horizontally not vertically. In other words, don't lick up and down the natural folds of the vulva. Lick across them. Go against the grain.

This provides a tremendously strong sensation for the clitoris because you are going back and forth across the sides of the clitoral hood, creating resistance and stimulation at the same time. This technique also puts you in a position where she can reach and rub your back and see more of your body.

23. Take her to the Top while on the Bottom

By far the best sexual position for strong female orgasm is Woman on Top or its backward cousin – the Reverse Cowgirl. In the Woman on Top position the man lies down and the woman straddles his body, taking his penis into her vaginal opening and creating friction by moving her hips up and down on his shaft.

It is a good position for climax because the angle of the penis hits the deeply sensitive front wall of the vaginal canal. It also serves to allow the female to control the speed, depth and thrusts so she can make sure she is hitting all the right spots. Woman on Top also allows you to face each other, so there is a lot of intimate eye contact. Depending on your height, you can also hold her hips or fondle her breasts as intercourse continues.

Reverse Cowgirl has the same elements only instead of facing the male partner the female straddles him and faces away from him. For some women who have body issues or simply don't like the vulnerability and exposure of the Woman on Top position, Reverse Cowgirl can make them feel more socially comfortable. At the same time, she is still able to control the level of penetration, speed and angle of the thrusts.

Reverse Cowgirl tends to generate less pressure on the front of the vaginal wall, but does provide more sensation to the pelvic floor and allow that area to tighten sufficiently for a powerful release. Both positions offer the benefit of allowing the female to reach down and stimulate her own clitoris while intercourse is occurring.

24. Who Let The Dogs Out?

Doggy style, otherwise known as "Rear Entry Vaginal Intercourse" is another fantastic position to use if giving your lover an amazing climax is one of your goals. Please note "rear entry" does not mean anal sex. This is a sexual position for vaginal sex.

Rear Entry Vaginal Intercourse can be achieved in a number of ways. The female partner bends over a bed (desk, couch arm, etc.) and the male partner stands behind her inserting his penis into her vaginally.

The other two popular methods are the "hands and knees" position where a woman gets on all fours and the male partner kneels behind her and penetrates her vaginally or the "face down/ass up" position where the woman is on her wrists or elbows and knees with her face as low to the carpet as it can go and her bottom sticking up. This allows the male partner to kneel or stand during rear entry.

All three variations of the doggy style position encourage deep penetration because of the straightening of the vaginal channel, and allow the penis to rub against the top of the vaginal wall (where the "G-spot" or erogenous zone is located) and push against the pelvic floor (where all the muscle tension happens).

Best of all, the position offers a good opportunity for the male partner to "reach around" the waist of his lover and use his hands to provide clitoral stimulation while simultaneously rocking back and forth in her body.

For strong orgasms and comfortable sex, doggy style can't be beat.

25. Do the Twist

A less well known sexual position for providing strong climax in women is the Twist. This position is best done on a bed or sleeping mat. In the Twist the female partner begins by lying flat on her back. The male partner lies beside her on his side facing her. The female then twists her hips and drapes her legs, slightly open, over the man's thighs. He penetrates her vaginally and the two rock together in a slow back and forth rhythm. It won't take long for her orgasm to ensue.

The secret of the Twist is the juxtaposition between the tight angle of his penis in her vagina and the openness and availability of the rest of her body. The position causes the penis to enter the vaginal at a nearly 30 degree angle, positioning the thrust up against the front vaginal wall. The angle of the legs/hips means her pelvic area is "locked in tight" which increases the muscle tension on the pelvic floor.

Because you two end up facing each other, you will have access to her breasts if you want to suck or fondle them, and can also use your hands to stimulate her clitoris. She can rub your chest, see your eyes or even engage in kissing as intercourse proceeds.

The Twist is an intimate, physically dynamic sexual position that is definitely worth a try.

26. Pillow talk

One of the best tools to keep on hand for maintaining proper positions and generating the kind of pulsing orgasm that will drive her wild is a pillow. Whether or not you are on a bed, using a pillow can definitely put her body at the right angle.

For sexual positions where she is on her back (traditional missionary position and its many variations) placing a pillow under her bottom lifts her hips at a 15 to 25 degree angle. This creates a more direct line for the penis to line up with the vaginal channel. The pillow also absorbs some of the pressure of the thrusts which takes the pressure off the lower back and hips.

For rear entry positions, having a pillow under her tummy or pelvic area takes the pressure off of the pelvic bone and lifts her bottom allowing for easier entry. Lifting her body in that scenario also lets gravity do its work as the penis moves downward and forward, providing the most natural entry and smooth rocking motion. Pillows can be placed behind her back to cushion the lower spine, or between her knees to keep her hips aligned and prevent cramping.

No matter where you make love, be sure to have a pillow or two around to be brought into action.

27. Use the CAT

For couples who have religious ideas, traditional understandings or simply don't want to use any other position than the missionary position (woman flat on her back, man on top of her holding himself up on his arms as he pushes forward) there is still a technique that can help her build to an outstanding climax. That technique is known as the CAT – Coital Alignment Technique. The CAT is often thought of as the missionary position with a bonus.

To begin with the male partner is on top of the woman and penetrates her vaginally, but just with the tip or first inch of the penis. He then moves forward lining his penis up so the base of his penis is pressing against her clitoris. Instead of thrusting, the couple rocks back and forth keeping constant pressure on the woman's clit.

The female gets the sensation of penetration and clitoral stimulation at the same time. Penetration is not deep, and this position is not recommended for women trying to get pregnant. Women who require more clitoral attention than vaginal find this position works extremely well.

Conclusion

Overall, as with all things that have to do with women and sex, the first and best thing to do is communicate with your partner.

Women who are sexually aware of their bodies will know exactly what works for them and where stimulation is best applied. Women who are less educated or experienced sexually may need you to teach them more about what their body can do under the right circumstances. Either way, talking and testing out difference sex position, techniques and styles is the best (and most fun) way to take this journey together. Let her teach you about her body but, rest assured, if you use some of the tips in this guide you will be teaching her as well.

Some of these techniques are as natural as turning on the coffee pot when you get up in the morning, and others will require a little practice. But, when it comes to providing your partner mind-blowing orgasms and increasing the sexual and psychological connection between you, practice doesn't just make perfect. Practice makes pleasure.

Books by Elizabeth Cramer:

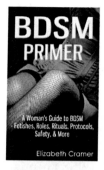

BDSM Primer - A Woman's Guide to BDSM - Fetishes, Roles, Rituals, Protocols, Safety, & More

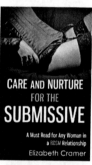

Care and Nurture for the Submissive - A Must Read for Any Woman in a BDSM Relationship

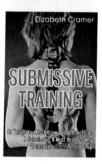

Submissive Training: 23 Things You Must Know About How To Be A Submissive. A Must Read For Any Woman In A BDSM Relationship

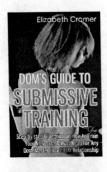
Dom's Guide To Submissive Training: Step-by-step Blueprint On How To Train Your New Sub. A Must Read For Any Dom/Master In A BDSM Relationship

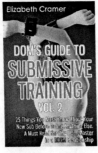
Dom's Guide To Submissive Training Vol. 2: 25 Things You Must Know About Your New Sub Before Doing Anything Else. A Must Read For Any Dom/Master In A BDSM Relationship

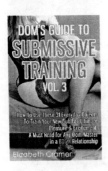
Dom's Guide To Submissive Training Vol. 3: How To Use These 31 Everyday Objects To Train Your New Sub For Ultimate Pleasure & Excitement. A Must Read For Any Dom/Master In A BDSM Relationship

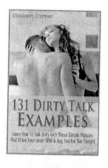

131 Dirty Talk Examples: Learn How To Talk Dirty with These Simple Phrases That Drive Your Lover Wild & Beg You For Sex Tonight

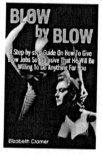

Blow By Blow - A Step-by-step Guide On How To Give Blow Jobs So Explosive That He Will Be Willing To Do Anything For You

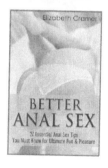

Better Anal Sex - 27 Essential Anal Sex Tips You Must Know for Ultimate Fun & Pleasure

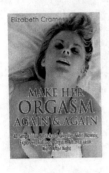

Make Her Orgasm Again and Again: 48 Simple Tips & Tricks to Give Her Mind-Blowing, Explosive, Full-Body Orgasm After Orgasm, Night After Night

CPSIA information can be obtained
at www.ICGtesting.com
Printed in the USA
FFOW04n1534141215
19650FF